Contents

Making Hair Color Complementary

Hair color at its best should be complementary to the individual. Factors to consider include:

Life style

The more outgoing the personality, the more exciting or dramatic your hair color result can be.

Facial shapes and features

Hair color should bring out the positive features and minimize any negative features.

Darker hair color can make features look smaller, while lighter hair color can make features look larger.

Examples are:

- A small face will appear larger with a lighter color of hair.

- Round, square, and full facial shapes will be minimized or complemented with darker colors.

- A pear shaped face will look best with a lighter hair color on the top of the head than the bottom.

Skin tone

- A warm sallow complexion will be complemented by gold and reds.

- A cool sallow complexion is complemented by gold, reds, and orange reds.

- A ruddy complexion needs to avoid ash or blue tones.

- An olive complexion is complemented by darker, deeper colors due to the depth of the skin tone. Dark cool tones and dark cool reds are also good.

The Five Steps to Fabulous Permanent Hair Color

To achieve a complementary hair color, it is important to complete five easy steps. The first four steps deal with achieving the best color formula, and the fifth step deals with choosing the correct volume of hydrogen peroxide (developer) necessary to achieve the color result.

Step 1. Determine the beginning level of hair color.

Step 2. Determine the desired level of hair color.

Step 3. Determine the desired tone of hair color.

Step 4. Determine the percentage of grey.

Step 5. Determine the correct hydrogen peroxide (developer).

Step 1: Determine the beginning level of hair color.

In order to fully understand the first step, we need to become familiar with the tool used to measure the beginning level of hair. We use a level system to determine where the hair is before you start the hair coloring process. We measure it from dark to light. Any head of hair will fall somewhere inside this level system.

Refer to figure I the Level System Chart (p.6). The Level System Chart begins at level 1 (the darkest level or black) and extends to level 10 (the lightest level).

The Level System Chart consists of the level numbers to the left. The level description is in the center, and the level measurement is to the right.

To determine your natural hair color level or the beginning level in your hair coloring process, select a section of hair close to the scalp. Compare that section to the colors on the color chart.

That color closest to your own hair color is the beginning level of hair to be colored. If you cannot decide between two levels, always choose the darker level.

Enter the beginning level number and description on the Fabulous Formulation Card on page 32 for Step 1.

I. Level System Chart		
#	**Description**	**Measurement**
10	Very light blonde	
9	Light blonde	
8	Medium blonde	
7	Dark blonde	
6	Light brown	
5	Medium brown	
4	Dark brown	
3	Very dark brown	
2	Black brown	
1	Black	

Step 2: Determine the desired level of hair color.

For Step 2, you need to determine your desired level of hair color. Throughout the rest of this manual, this desired level will be used to select the hair color product that will be applied to the hair, so give this answer special consideration. You are not selecting the actual color, just the level.

Using the Level System Chart (p.6), determine your desired level...one that will be complementary and flattering.

- Do you want your hair color to be lighter?

- Do you want your hair color to be your natural level?

- Do you want your hair color to be darker than your natural level?

Once you have selected your desired level, enter your level number and description on your Fabulous Formulation Card on page 32 for Step 2.

The Color Wheel

The Color Wheel (p. 9) is the most important part of the hair coloring process.

The outer ring of the Color Wheel is composed of the universal *primary colors* yellow, red, and blue.

The middle ring is composed of the *secondary colors* of orange, violet, and green. They are created by mixing two primary colors together.

The inner ring is composed of the *tertiary colors* yellow-orange, red-orange, red-violet, blue-violet, blue-green, and yellow-green. Tertiary colors are created by mixing a primary color with secondary color.

Now imagine a line drawn vertically through the center of the Color Wheel, cutting the Color Wheel in half.

The left side is dominated by warm colors such as red and yellow. Therefore, this side is considered the warm side of the Color Wheel.

The right side is dominated by cool colors such as blue and green. Therefore, this side is considered the cool side of the Color Wheel.

The center of the Color Wheel is a mixture of the three primary colors. Any time you mix these three primary colors together you will create brown.

The very center is *neutral,* not warm or cool.

II. The Color Wheel

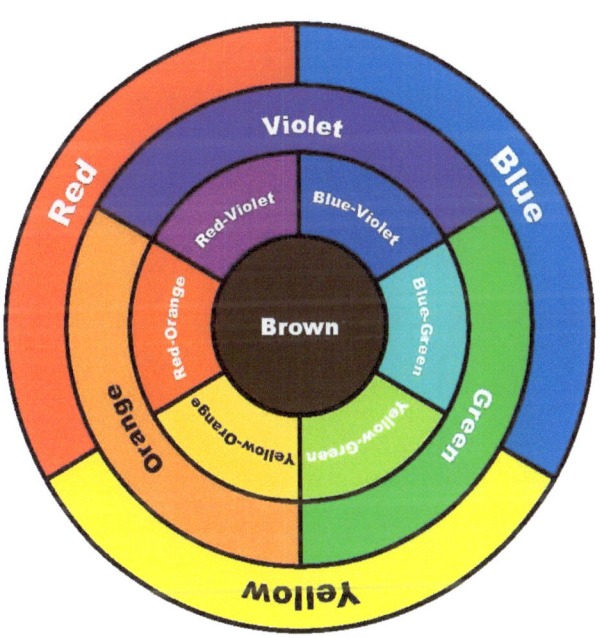

Warm side   Cool side

Step 3: Determine the desired tone.

Tone of hair color means the degree of warmth or coolness of color.

If your desired tone is dominated by red, yellow, or gold, the hair color will be considered warm. If your desired tone is dominated by blue or green, the hair color will be considered cool. If the hair is not warm or cool, it will be considered a *natural* tone or neutral. The center of the Color Wheel would be considered a *natural* tone.

To create a particular tone, we must also understand the Underlying Color Chart (p.11). The Underlying Color Chart consists of the level number to the left. The level description is in the center. The underlying color for each level is to the right.

The underlying color is the dominant color at each particular level.

For example, if your desired level of hair color is 4, then your underlying color will be red-violet.

What is the underlying color at your desired level?

Enter the underlying color at your desired level on your Fabulous Formulation Card on page 32 for Step 3.

III. The Underlying Color Chart

#	Level description	Underlying color
10	Very light blonde	Yellow-white
9	Light blonde	Yellow
8	Medium blonde	Yellow-orange
7	Dark blonde	Orange
6	Light brown	Red-orange
5	Medium brown	Red
4	Dark brown	Red-violet
3	Very dark brown	Violet
2	Black brown	Blue-violet
1	Black	blue

Now that we are familiar with the Underlying Color Chart, we can examine the hair coloring process and its effects on the underlying color.

Before we can fully understand the hair coloring process, we have to understand that all *natural* hair or virgin hair is a mixture of the three primary colors in proportionate amounts.

In the examples below, the bold primary color is the most dominate in theory.

Examples are as follows:

- Black/ brown hair consists of (red, yellow and dominate **blue**).

- Medium brown hair contains (blue, red and yellow).

- A natural red head is a red-brown which includes (blue, yellow and dominate **red**).

- A natural blonde is a yellow-brown and contains (blue, red and dominate **yellow**).

Natural or virgin hair is hair that has never had a permanent hair color product applied to it.

If all *natural* hair or virgin hair contains the three primary colors in proportionate amounts, then all *natural looking* hair color must also contain all three primary colors in proportionate amounts.

The Hair Coloring Process and Its Effects on Your Underlying Color:

When permanently coloring hair with a one step permanent hair color product, there are three things one can accomplish:

1) You can lighten the hair.

2) You can color at the same level.

3) You can darken the hair.

Lightening the hair

When the hair is lightened, the underlying color changes, you can follow along on your Underlying Color Chart (p.11) starting with blue at level 1.

When you lighten the hair

- The blue primary will leave the hair first.

- Next, the red will leave the hair.

- Then, yellow will leave the hair.

- Finally, the hair will lose all of the primary, secondary, and tertiary color. The hair is left white.

The color left in the hair after the lightening process is complete is called the **underlying color.**

You cannot lighten the hair more than three to four levels with a one-step permanent hair color product. It is very important to understand that if the hair has been previously colored with a one-step permanent hair color product; it cannot be lightened predictably using a one-step permanent hair color product. However, it can be colored level-on-level or darker.

Coloring at the same level

When coloring at the same level, the desired level is the same as the beginning level. It is important to know what the underlying color is for your desired level because that is the level you will be coloring the hair.

Darkening the hair

When darkening the hair, the end result will be darker than the beginning level of hair color. It is important to be aware of the underlying color or tone of your beginning level.

This is where the Color Wheel becomes very important in creating great hair color. Think about this statement.

The underlying hair color mixed with any base color will determine the remaining hair color.

Your remaining hair color result can be achieved using the Color Wheel in these three ways:

1) You can work opposite the underlying color on the Color Wheel.

2) You can work around the Color Wheel using your underlying color.

3) You can work opposite and around the Color Wheel at the same time.

Mixing opposites on the Color Wheel

In this information, when I refer to a *natural* result, it simply means a balance of blue, red, and yellow at any given level of hair color.

When you mix colors opposite on the Color Wheel equally, the end result will be a *natural brown* because you are mixing all three primary colors together.

1

Draw a line from blue through the center of the wheel to orange (red and yellow).

Blue + orange (yellow and red) = *natural brown*

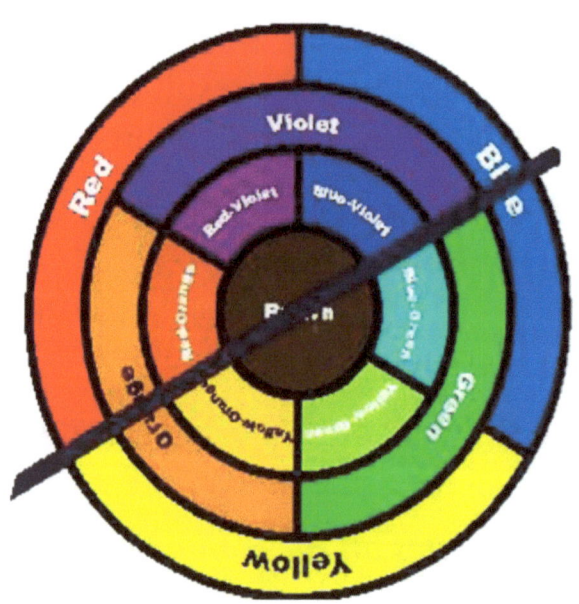

If you mix blue with orange (yellow + red), you are mixing all three primary colors. Mixed together they would create *natural brown*.

Draw a line from yellow through the center of the color wheel to violet (red and blue).

Yellow + violet (red + blue) = *natural brown*

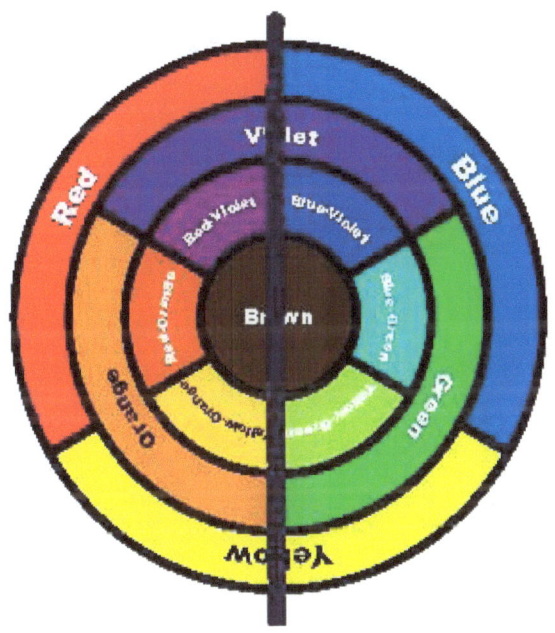

If you mix yellow with violet (red + blue), you are mixing all three primary colors. Mixed together they will create *natural brown*.

Working around the Color Wheel

Select red-orange from the Color Wheel.

Red-orange + orange = orange red-orange

If you mix red-orange with orange, the end result is orange red-orange.

Select red from the Color Wheel.

Red + violet = red-violet

If you mix red with violet, the end result is red-violet.

Select violet from the Color Wheel.

Violet + green = red-brown

If you mix Violet (red + blue) with green (blue + yellow), the end result is cool red brown.

Working opposite and around at the same time

Select red-orange from the Color Wheel.

Red-orange + blue-green = *natural brown*

To create *natural brown,* you must look at the Color Wheel and determine that blue-green is directly opposite of red-orange. Mixed together they would create *natural brown.*

Red-orange + blue-green = *natural red-brown*

+ Violet

What if you wanted a red brown?

If you mix red-orange + blue-green + a cool red such as violet, the end result is red-brown.

Select yellow-orange from the Color Wheel.

Yellow-orange + blue-violet = *natural medium*

blonde

To create *natural medium blond,* you must look at the Color Wheel and determine that blue-violet is directly opposite of yellow-orange. Mixed together they would create *natural medium blonde.*

What if you wanted a cool blonde?

Yellow-orange + blue-violet = *natural medium*
+ Blue *cool blonde*

If you mix yellow-orange + blue-violet + blue (cool), the end result will be *natural medium cool blonde.*

It is that simple. Natural looking hair color results are based on the theory that opposites on the Color Wheel create brown.

We can, however, use a portion of our formula to create a *natural* result and a portion to add a particular tone to the hair.

What is your desired level?

What is the underlying color at your desired level?

What is directly opposite from your underlying color on the Color Wheel?

Enter the opposite color of your underlying color on you Fabulous Formulation Card on page 32 for Step 3.

Step 4: Determine the percentage of grey.

In Step 4, we need to determine approximately how much grey is in our *natural* hair to ensure a pleasant result from our hair-color service.

The reason we must do this is that grey hair does not contain the *natural* balance of blue, red, and yellow. Therefore, the grey hair should be considered to be white, an absence of color.

One way to compensate for the grey is to use a *natural* color equal to the percentage of grey in the hair. A *natural* base color contains a balance of blue, red, and yellow. All hair color companies have a *natural* base color available at each level.

There are three situations we need to consider when covering grey:

1) Covering grey below 50%.

2) Covering grey 50% or above.

3) Covering grey level 5 and darker.

Covering grey under 50 percent

When there is less than fifty percent grey in your *natural* hair, that percentage of grey hair must be compensated for by using a *natural* base color equal to the percentage of grey hair. A *natural* base color contains a balance of blue, red and yellow.

Example:

Your hair contains 30% grey. Your desired level of color is a level 6 light *natural brown*. Checking III, The Underlying Color Chart (p.11), you see that your underlying color at level 6 is red-orange

Red-orange + blue-green = *natural brown*

To create *natural brown* (with no grey), you look at the Color Wheel and determine that blue-green is directly opposite of red-orange. Mixed together these colors will create *natural brown* at level 6.

With 30% grey our new formula would be:

Red-orange + 70% blue-green = *natural brown*

+ *30% light brown*

70% blue-green (to create brown with red-orange underlying color) and 30% *natural* base color to compensate for the grey.

Covering grey over 50 percent

When covering grey more than fifty percent, the largest part of the hair does not contain any primary color (blue, red or yellow). Therefore, all three primary colors must be added to the hair for a *natural* looking hair color result.

Example:

The hair contains 100 percent grey. Your desired level of color is a level 8 *natural medium blonde*. In this example, the underlying color is considered white.

3 parts *natural medium blonde* (blue, red & yellow)

1 part red medium blonde (red)

1 part golden medium blonde (yellow)

If you were to mix three parts *natural medium blonde*, one part medium red blonde and one part medium golden blonde. You are mixing all three primary colors. The end result would be *natural medium blonde* at level 8.

Covering grey at level 5 or darker

When covering grey at level 5 or darker, it is recommended that you use one level of color lighter than your desired level. (Most people perceive their *natural* level of hair to be lighter if it contains grey.)

Once you have selected your percentage of grey, enter it on your Fabulous Formulation Card on page 32 for Step 4.

Step 5: Determine the correct volume of hydrogen peroxide (developer).

In Step 5, you need to determine the correct hydrogen peroxide (developer) needed to lighten or to darken the hair to the desired level.

Look at your Fabulous Formulation Card on page 33 of this manual.

- Is your desired level lighter than your beginning level? How many levels lighter?

  Note: You cannot lighten the hair more than three to four levels with a one step permanent hair color product.

- Is your desired level the same as your beginning level of color?

- Is your desired level darker than your beginning level of color?

When your desired level is darker than your natural level with very little grey, you may need only a 15 volume hydrogen peroxide (developer). Choose the correct hydrogen peroxide (developer) from the Hydrogen Peroxide Chart below.

IV. HYDROGEN PEROXIDE CHART

Level on level or darker	15 - 20 volume peroxide
One level lighter	20 volume hydrogen peroxide
Two levels lighter	30 volume hydrogen peroxide
Three to four levels lighter	40 volume hydrogen peroxide

Once you have selected your desired hydrogen peroxide (developer), enter it on your Fabulous Formulation Card on page 32 Step 5.

Applications

When applying hair color to the hair, it is important to consider how the product will be applied to the hair in order to accomplish an even hair color result throughout the entire head of hair.

There are two types of applications:

Virgin Application-Hair has not been previously permanently colored with a one-step permanent hair color product.

- Apply ½ inch away from scalp.
- Process the color ½ the processing time.
- Then apply to roots and ends.
- Process the color the original full processing time.

Retouch Application-Hair has been previously permanently colored with a one-step permanent hair color product.

- Apply to root area

- If pulling through, add ½ ounce of water to color formula

- If the color formula contains warm tones (Red or gold), add 1/5 ounce of that warm tone to color formula before pulling through ends

- Pull through ends the last ten to twenty minutes when ends need refreshed (every second to third application)

This manual should be used as a guide in the one-step permanent hair coloring processes. The process consists of formulation, selection, and application, in that order.

The Five Steps to Fabulous Permanent Hair Color will be used for formulation. The Fabulous Formulation Card on page 33 will be used as a guide to selecting the one-step permanent hair color product at the point of purchase.

To correctly select the appropriate hair color product, you will need to know these four things.

1) The desired level,

2) The desired tone,

3) The percentage of grey, and

4) The correct hydrogen peroxide(developer).

The desired level

All permanent hair color products are labeled with the level of hair color they are designed to achieve.

Hair color companies use similar level systems. Familiarize yourself with their systems if needed.

The desired tone

When selecting a one-step permanent hair color product, you will need to know the base or bases of color you need to apply for your desired tone.

The underlying hair color mixed with any base color will determine the remaining hair color.

Many permanent hair color products contain brown bases with the addition of a particular tone.

Pay close attention to the tone of hair color you are purchasing.

- Blue green = ash

- Blue violet = natural

- Red = red

- Yellow = gold

The percentage of grey

You should also know the percentage of grey so that you can compensate for its missing primary colors by using a *natural* base color equal to the percentage of grey.

Most hair color companies have a *natural* base color available at each level.

The correct hydrogen peroxide

Most pre-packaged one step permanent hair color products only contain a 20 volume hydrogen peroxide (developer). If a larger volume is needed, you will have to purchase it separately from a beauty supply and mix it in equal parts with the hair color itself.

It is very important to understand that hair color companies can label their one-step permanent hair color products differently.

To be successful when selecting a one-step permanent hair color product, you must familiarize yourself with the hair color product you are going to use.

Most point-of-purchase outlets have tools available to familiarize you with the hair-color products available.

If it is necessary to use more than one bottle or tube of hair color in your hair color formula, you will need to purchase a clear bottle that is labeled in increments of ounces, or a bowl and brush to mix in.

Most one-step permanent hair-color products are mixed equal parts hair color to equal parts hydrogen peroxide (developer).

About the author

Adam Casteel has been a professional hair stylist for over twenty six years. He is an expert in the art and science of hair color.

However, Adam noticed there is a lack of information about the hair coloring process for individuals and stylist alike.

In this manual, Adam shares the best basic hair coloring theory. He has used his education, knowledge, and expertise to make the art of hair coloring easy and rewarding for the reader.

His Five Steps to Fabulous Hair Color will help produce beautiful hair and provide you with confidence to be more successful in your hair-coloring process. It will take the guess work out of the hair-coloring process and help you accomplish a more pleasing result each and every time you use it.

3

Fabulous Formulation Card

Step 1	Determine your natural level	
Step 2	Determine your desired level	
Step 3	Determine the desired tone of your end result by finding:	
	(A) Underlying color at the desired level	
	(B) Opposite of underlying on color wheel	
Step 4	Determine the correct hydrogen peroxide.	
Step 5	Determine the percentage of gray.	

Disclaimer: This is only a guide to successful hair color. The results may vary depending on the hair to be colored.

The provider of this information is in no way responsible for any results that may come from the application of hair color to any head of hair.

Five Steps to Fabulous Hair color
Adam Casteel
Copyright# TXu-1-656-097